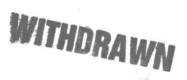

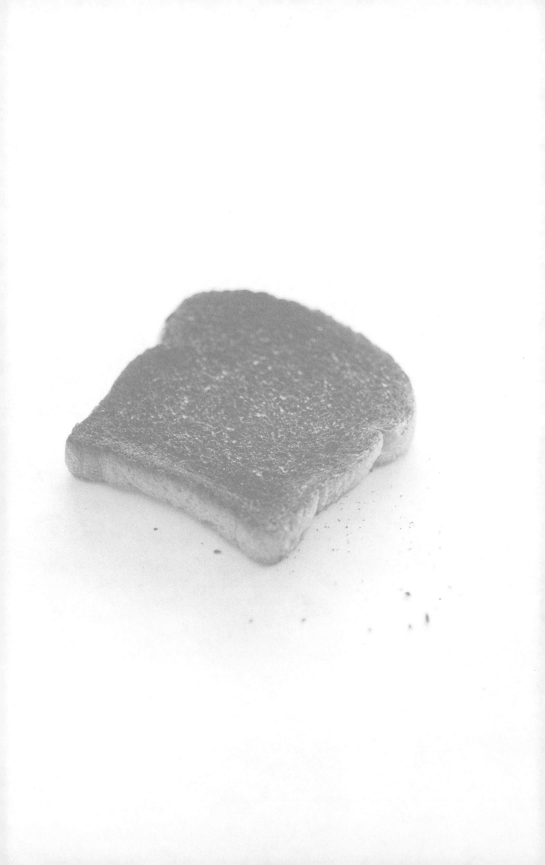

GLUTEN

is my

BITCH

GLUTEN
is my
BITCH

Rants, Recipes, and
RIDICULOUSNESS
for the
Gluten-Free

April Peveteaux

Stewart, Tabori & Chang | New York

Published in 2013 by Stewart, Tabori & Chang
An imprint of ABRAMS

Library of Congress Cataloging-in-Publication Data
Peveteaux, April.
  Gluten is my bitch : recipes, rants, and ridiculousness for the gluten-free / April Peveteaux.
    pages cm
   ISBN 978-1-61769-030-3 (hardback)
1. Gluten-free diet—Recipes. 2. Gluten-free foods. 3. Comfort food.
I. Title.
 RM237.86.P48 2013
 641.5'63—dc23
                         2013006605

Editor: Jennifer Levesque
Designer: Rachel Willey
Production Manager: True Sims

The text of this book was composed in Garamond, Nobel, and Freehand 575 BT.

Printed and bound in the U.S.A.
10 9 8 7 6 5 4 3 2 1

Stewart, Tabori & Chang books are available at special discounts when purchased in quantity for premiums and promotions as well as fund-raising or educational use. Special editions can also be created to specification. For details, contact specialsales@abramsbooks.com or the address below.

ABRAMS
THE ART OF BOOKS SINCE 1949

115 West 18th Street
New York, NY 10011
www.abramsbooks.com

For Mom.
(Sorry for all the cursing.)

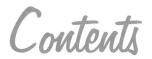

Contents

Introduction

Are you perusing the "special diet" section of the bookstore right now, picking up gluten-free tomes and trying to figure out if this is the book that will be useful in your gluten-free quest (or forcible life sentence)? Let me go ahead and answer that question for you: It totally will.

I'm guessing you're looking for a little guidance, maybe some crazy delicious recipes, and a whole lot of poop jokes. You've come to the right place. But wait, there's more! I'm also here to offer you hope. Hope that someday you will feel normal again, and be able to go back to avoiding any section in the bookstore that uses the word "health" as a descriptor. Hope that even though you're giving up gluten now, you can still enjoy devil's food cake. Maybe even hope that, while you go about the business of discovering what is up with gluten-free doughnuts, a REAL doughnut might be in your future. Just wait until I tell you what medical science is up to in celiac research. Yeah, it is awesome, and I'm stoked to take you on this journey to Hopesville.

You may be wondering why I am spending my time trying to make you—the gluten intolerant—feel better about your current situation. That is a very good question, my brand-new and incredibly good-looking friend.

It was only a few years ago when I found myself in your position; wondering how I had fallen so far from being the "new fiction" browser in the store to now standing in front of the diet section looking for answers to questions about my jacked-up digestion. Sure, I was able to score some great books filled with gluten-free recipes and a few celebrity-penned tales of gluten gone wrong. Yet what I really needed was someone to tell me it was going to be all right. Not "It's going to be great! Why don't you go ahead and cut out dairy, casein, sugar, and all fun?" Instead, wondering why no one else seemed pissed off about this situation, I left the bookstore with another Swedish mystery in hand and an incredible sense of inferiority about my bad gluten-free attitude.

Just like your therapist would tell you, sometimes you have to be your own BFF. I went home and created my blog, Gluten Is My Bitch, and started talking big-time smack about gluten and the celiac disease that had suddenly appeared and taken away my villi. It helped. It really helped when I started experimenting with my deep-fat fryer, and even more so when people seemed to enjoy learning how to make gluten-free cakes, pies, and cookies as much as I enjoyed eating the creations. And that's why this book is sitting in your hands. The gluten-free people want to eat cake. The fact is, more and more people are going gluten-free and all of them aren't into mixing twenty-eight flours to make the perfect soufflé, or chanting "I'm Grateful" while they dine out. Those people need some Gluten Is My Bitch in their lives. Just like you do!

Let's bring it down for just a minute. Here's the thing about going gluten-free, whether you've been given a celiac disease diagnosis or just know you feel better when you're not enjoying cinnamon rolls for breakfast, flatbread pizza for lunch, and a pile of spaghetti Bolognese for dinner: It's fucking hard. I won't sugarcoat that for you, so if you're looking for a book to cheerlead you all the way to Vegantown, maybe look up and to your left. (Note: I do have some amazing gluten-free and vegan recipes inside these pages, 'cuz I'm all-inclusive like that.) Smiling through the pain of watching your friends enjoy unlimited breadsticks while your plate sits empty does not change the intensity of our shared gluten-free torment. Let's own that pain and complain about it until we're asked to leave the party. It's not all about wallowing in self-pity, though plenty of that is certainly in order. You are giving up chocolate croissants, after all.

Gluten Is My Bitch: Rants, Recipes, and Ridiculousness for the Gluten-Free will try a little bit to make you see the bright side, but if you don't want to, I won't dismiss you as "difficult" and will instead take you out for tequila shots (naturally gluten-free, y'all!) and tacos. I'll also tell you plenty of off-color jokes on the way to conquering your gluten-free diet, and hold your hair when you throw up. We are a unique people who cannot enjoy the best of what the bakery has to offer any longer, and so therefore we deserve special treatment, yet no one really wants to give it to us. But I will. In fact, I am! I'm ready to pamper you and poke with a stick anyone who dares get in my way. That's just the kind of gal I am.

Perhaps, before delving into *Gluten Is My Bitch*, you would like to see some credentials. How about I ask the same of you? As someone who knows how to use the hell out of Google, I will now diagnosis you based on symptoms and Internet searches. Those of you who discover through my incredibly nonprofessional quiz that you are, indeed, gluten intolerant are welcome. The rest of you are welcome too, but you should really see someone about that gout. Ready? Answer me this:

1. When I wake up in the morning:

a) I have to throw up.
b) My sheets feel like they are slicing my big toe into a million pieces.
c) My energy is at its highest and I jump out of bed, excited to begin a new day.
d) I'm still tired.

2. After lunch, I usually:

a) Feel good for the first time all day, at least until I get hungry half an hour later.
b) Wonder what's up with my throbbing big toe.
c) Hit the gym—it's the best time to take advantage of my post-lunch energy boost.
d) Poop my pants.

3. The last thing I think about before I go to sleep is:

a) Is it too early to have breakfast?
b) Is it okay to wear ski boots to bed, on account of this pain in my toe that is aggravated by my sheets?
c) I had the most amazing day and I feel GREAT!
d) Wow, I sure am . . . zzzzzzzz . . .

If you answered *a* on every question: Congratulations, you're pregnant!
If you answered *b* on every question: Damn, son, you've got the gout.
If you answered *c* on every question: I fucking hate you.
If you answered *d* on every question: Yep, you've got a gluten problem.

For all of you "d" people, come join me in the gluten-free world as I continue to make new discoveries, with much emphasis on the ridiculousness of our shared bread-free situation. Really, it's OK in here. I mean, not as OK as eating brioche every day for breakfast, but it'll do. Welcome.

Chapter One

WHAT TO DO WHEN YOU'RE
Crapping Your Pants

Hello there! If you picked up this book because you're crapping your pants, I have to say you've come to the right place. So pull up your bowl and squat because I can fill you in on what funny things are happening to your body. Almost as uncomfortable as "the talk" we're going to go through your digestive system and work out what this crazy problem actually is, or is not. Most likely you're blaming gluten right about now because, come on, *it's the worst.* Do you have the autoimmune disorder celiac disease? (Note: If you're European, it's coeliac or the very cutely named, "sprue." Lucky Europeans.) Do you have a wheat allergy? Or are you one of those illusive "gluten intolerants"? Maybe you've decided it's about time you tried that paleo diet all the kids are talking about. Whatever your gluten situation, you're probably here because there is pooping, or perhaps, retching involved. If you're super lucky you'll also have a little itchiness, a bit of achiness, or all around crankiness. Which means it's time to start making some incredibly painful and permanent choices about the most important thing in your life, which is, of course, food. If you thought it was something else, perhaps you should look at a different book, like say, *The Secret.* But if you're here to learn about your weird physical ailments, read on my disgusting friends.

So, what seems to be the problem? Check one:

 I am bloated, gassy, and no fun to be around.

 I have a rash that won't go away. No, it's not syphilis. Stop looking at me that way.

 I'm so tired I've given up on the disco nap and just take a pre-bedtime nap.

 I'm pretty sure I'm allergic to turkey, rather than the delicious sourdough it is served upon. Stupid turkey.

 Between the brain fog and the creaky joints, I've turned into that old guy who screams at empty chairs.

 I'm losing a scary amount of weight, and it's really not awesome anymore.

Or perhaps, you, like me, had violent diarrhea for three months straight, wound up in the hospital, and finally decided to take control of your digestive situation.

We are a fun bunch, are we not?

No matter what kind of sickness has taken hold of you, let's blame gluten. If you want or need to get gluten out of your diet, bravo! Kick that nasty gluten to the curb, I say. Pretend it's an unwanted cat (which I'm also allergic to, so *no problem*), or that one ex-partner who is such a mistake you still cringe when you think about being seen with him/her. What were you thinking? Really?

But before you totally and completely ban wheat, barley, rye, and the odd man out—triticale—you should consider the following:

- Maybe it really *is* the turkey.

- Perhaps you just have pinworms. In which case, whew! (And please never sleep over at my house.)

- I hate to even bring this up, but it could be the dairy.

- You've been watching too much *Grey's Anatomy* and are self-diagnosing without a medical degree or improv classes.

- You don't realize beer and cake both have gluten.

After contemplating all of the above, and more, you still may want to cut gluten out of your diet. I'm not here to discourage you but simply to make sure you totally get that gluten tastes awesome, and you should seriously consider what your life would look like without gluten. (It will look cake-less and beer-less, FYI.) But if you've been diagnosed with celiac disease, or you're one of the twenty million Americans stricken with gluten sensitivity, it's time to kick some gluten ass—and read this book.

Not sure if gluten-free is for you? Perhaps gluten simply causes you some discomfort, but you've never been diagnosed. Then eff that gluten! Get it out of your system, ban it from your cupboard, and kick it out, with my help. The fact is, gluten sensitivity can be damn tricky to diagnosis, even though your symptoms are the same—or worse—than those of your friend who looks totally legit, what with her celiac disease diagnosis. Don't let anyone tell you it's all in your head because even if it *is* all in your head, it's still coming out of your rear parts. If something is making you sick, stay away from it, no matter how tempting. That includes beer and cake, dammit.

Listen, some people will make you feel bad for wanting to disrespect gluten. After all, bread is the staff of life and all that. Some of us with celiac disease might think you're just trying to be trendy, and you could possibly hurt our reputation. Personally, my reputation is already shot the minute I walk into a restaurant and identify myself as having special needs—so I'm cool with all that. If you don't want gluten in your life, send it packing. Honestly, no matter which way you come to gluten-free, I will not judge. I will, however, feel super stoked to have a meal with you so I won't be the only weirdo at the table.

For those of you who have been suffering in silence, or suffering loudly and obnoxiously; or those who have suddenly found yourselves getting sick every time you grab lunch at the fried-chicken palace; or even those who just like reading scatological nonfiction—welcome. No matter why you're here, I'm going to help you out and off the pot. Or at least, help you laugh while you're on the pot. Which is really how all great works should be measured: Does it keep me entertained whilst on the pot?

I realize that some of you are incredibly angry right now. Those of you with small children with celiac are ready to punch a doctor then cry yourself to sleep for the next six months. It's true that this is a crappy situation. But we can get through it together, if only we make fun of it and learn how to eat Buffalo wings again without getting violently ill. That's a laudable goal, for us gluten-haters. You may not feel like you're ready to laugh yet, but I say you are. Since I am the boss of this book, you must obey or have a time out while you think about your actions.

Ready? Even if—out of a strict sense of duty or gravity—you insist on keeping your laugh lines perfectly straight throughout the reading of this guide, I'm still going to help you conquer that devil gluten. Exorcise it from your life, and your gut, and replace it with much better options, as well as lots of confidence when you head out to dinner. No more contemplating adult diapers or resorting to wearing your old granny panties on dinner dates. This no-bullshit guide is going to allow you to live loud, proud, and gluten-free.

Who the Heck Are You?

You may be thinking, "Hey, April has celiac disease. Why is she so dang happy? How does she stay so Zen when she can't order off the menu anymore without harassing the entire waitstaff and the chef? How is it she can laugh about this whole gluten-free diet suckage when it does, indeed, suck so much?"

Here's the thing. First of all, it's an angry laugh. Plus, I've had a little bit of time to work through my deprivation issues and gluten challenges. I was once like you: just waking up from anesthesia and finding out that "Waffle Wednesdays" are now a thing of the past. Sure I was angry, peeved, and petulant. But then I realized how to be totally, 100 percent OK with cutting gluten out of my diet. It's absolutely no problem to go gluten-free as long *as everyone else in the entire world does it too.*

Since it seems like this is the way people are going, well, we celiacs have really won this war, don't you think? Approximately three million Americans have celiac disease, and probably two million poor saps are going around without knowing they are part of the club: pooping, crying, and wondering what the heck is going on with their digestive system. *There are twenty million of us who are gluten intolerant.* That's a huge amount of people clamoring for gluten-free goods! There are athletes, celebrities, and crazy people, all demanding gluten-free food be shoved into their gullets. Which is actually great for us celiac types because now we can walk into French Laundry and get gluten-free bread. Wendy's offers a gluten-free menu—some of the gluten-free foodstuffs even qualify as "value." We've won! Now, don't you feel better? No? Darn it; are you still bloated and irritable? OK, then, let's get real.

How Do You Know If Gluten Is Really the One?

Just like your latest Internet date, it can be difficult to figure out if gluten is the one you should never, ever see or talk to or breathe upon again. The fact of the matter is that celiacs take an average of ten years[1] to get diagnosed. So you may be going around crapping your pants for a very long time and hearing doctors tell you that it's all in your head or that you're just "stressed." Of course you're stressed: YOU'RE CRAPPING YOUR PANTS. Because there is no test for the gluten intolerant, you guys just have to figure this business out for yourselves. With the average diagnosis of celiac disease taking so

---

1 Six to ten years is the average time a person waits to be correctly diagnosed. (Source: Daniel Leffler, M.D., M.S., The Celiac Center at Beth Israel Deaconness Medical Center.)

damn long, and no quick way to alert the gluten sensitive, you can understand why so many celiacs and intolerants are kind of downers. That's ten years (or more!) of doctors telling you to go home and eat more yogurt. I can't even imagine what it would be like to be sick for ten years with no diagnosis. Which is why I consider myself extremely lucky to have gotten violently ill continuously until I had to admit that the only option was to have someone knock me out and shove something up my butt and down my throat.

Which brings us to how you know you have celiac disease. Celiac disease can be diagnosed in a few different ways, but the proof is in the villi. You know, those hairy-looking things in your small intestine that suck up all the vitamins and nutrients your body needs to function? If you have the auto-immune disease of celiac, you can say good-bye to those cute little villi. In fact, mine were completely gone. Or as my gastroenterologist said, "It looks like someone took an axe to your villi." Nice violent imagery there, but I'm pretty sure he felt he had to get brutal with someone who let her body become completely worn down without picking up the phone to call a doctor until she wound up in the emergency room. The good news is, if your villi are gone, your doctor can tell you with confidence that you have celiac disease.[2]

The bad news is, your villi are gone and you have celiac disease. But yet again, the good news is, I'm totally going to help you figure out how to live without gluten. Hooray, me! Hooray, you! Boo, gluten!

If you went straight for the endoscopy and learned about your villi situation, you're good, as well as a total badass. But if you want to start slowly, perhaps your first step toward celiac diagnosis will involve a tissue transglutaminase antibody test, which is also known as the tTG test. This test shows if you have antibodies that are consistent with celiac disease. Maybe your blood test came back positive for celiac disease. Hey, mine did too! But the blood test also came back positive for Crohn's disease, which is a heck of a lot scarier than celiac. (If you're Crohn's and gluten-free, welcome! I love your kind and have nothing but respect for those of you who aren't just, like, "Fuck it,

---

2 I am so totally not a doctor. I just write books about disgusting medical conditions. Please consult your doctor for a proper diagnosis.

take out my intestines so I can eat biscuits and gravy." Hell, I have respect for those of you who *do* say that. Mad respect.) So this is why the biopsy via endoscopy is always a fantastic idea in order to get an accurate diagnosis.

If you haven't been offered this biopsy option, you need to get serious with your doctor. Although I was rushed into the endoscopy and colonoscopy option, I've heard horror stories of people who were ignored by their doctors, never taken seriously when they complained of aches, pains, rashes, diarrhea, vomiting, and all-around unwellness. If you find yourself in a doctor's office with an unresponsive physician, you've got to be loud and *demand* a diagnosis. Celiac is no joke, nor is any food allergy or intolerance. They may be easy to make fun of, but if you don't have celiac under control, it can be

Craziest Things I've Said While Suffering a Gluten Attack

1. Here, take this Ziploc bag of poop to the emergency room and have them analyze it.

2. I know I said before that if I died, I didn't want you to re-marry, but now that I think it's going to happen, do what you've got to do.

3. I really don't think it was the gluten.

4. Can you please go get me a skinny vanilla latte?

5. I'm fine.

life threatening. I'll get into all the awesome diseases undiagnosed celiac can bring on later, but right now we're only talking about pleasant things. Like how I found out I could no longer visit The Grilled Cheese Truck when it was so thoughtfully parked in the Frosted Cupcakery parking lot.

About Me and My Disgusting, Disgusting Body

Not surprisingly, my digestive issues began shortly after I moved to Los Angeles. Also not surprisingly, I blamed everything on my cross-country move as I left behind my beloved Brooklyn, along with all of my street cred. But I had a family now, and one must do what's best for the children, and that meant moving somewhere with perfect weather and employment opportunities for the man who makes the real money in our household—my husband. After all, I'm just a writer, and we all know how the Internet has ruined all of our chances of ever making money again. So thank you for buying this book and allowing me to purchase my very expensive gluten-free saltines. You may also need to get a second job (or write a book, 'cuz you know, it's *super easy*) in order to afford all of those new gluten-free foods. But we'll explore that later, when I take you on a journey through the supermarket.

Back to the pooping and Los Angeles. Like I said, I was ripped from Brooklyn and plopped down in Southern California, where I worked from home and shuttled my kids around to day care and preschool. Every now and then I would find myself in debilitating pain and hanging out on the pot all day. As someone who had previously eaten Mexican food and barbecue at every single meal, I was shocked at my sudden delicate constitution. Yet I ignored it. Or rather, tried to work around it.

And everything would have been fine had it not been for my husband and his love of not having a heart attack in his thirties. Suddenly the man I married had the genius idea that we should try to go vegetarian for a month. Give it the old college try, since hey, we'd done it for an entire week a few years ago and that worked out *not at all* well. Why not go for an entire month of getting creative in the kitchen, which also translates to buying things in packages and reheating? Here's how it all went horribly wrong: You know what vegetarians eat, right? Gluten. Those people eat tons and tons of gluten. You've got your seitan and your pasta, your couscous, and lots of grilled cheese sandwiches. And this is why I can blame my celiac disease on vegetarianism and/or my husband.

Instead of feeling light and airy and super smug about not eating meat, I instead found myself in a constant state of beshatting. Still, I was blaming my move, my stressful job, and the lack of insulation in our rental home (seriously, California, get it together). For a moment I even blamed my best friend, dairy. But that didn't last long because I really couldn't stay mad at dairy. Can anyone? In hindsight, I'd had a few severe bouts of stomach distress in the previous year, and I was convinced that I had developed arthritis at a very young age. Then there was that whole winter in New York when I thought the cold was responsible for my dry, flaky skin, yet it did not change even when I visited Texas, the land of humidity and the burrito. So even though the vegetarianism put me totally over the edge, the celiac symptoms had been slowly sneaking up, ready to attack as soon as they had a great reason. That great reason was pasta every day for a month.

It wasn't until I wound up in the emergency room because I was pretty sure my stomach was about to rip out of my body, and I couldn't even breathe through the pain, that I finally took some advice from the ER doc. Two months later I walked into my fantastic GI doctor's office (I know! How stubborn am I?) and was quickly scheduled for an endoscopy and colonoscopy.

If you've never had the joy of a procedure that requires you empty out your entire insides before even stepping inside the doctor's office, you are missing out on a serious good time. Yet here's how sick I had been up until that point: When it was my turn to drink that battery acid that clears out your entire digestive system for, like, two days, it didn't even faze me. Yep, my daily living with explosive diarrhea was much worse than the colon blow most people avoid even at the cost of dying from cancer. I remember coming out of the bathroom at midnight after about sixteen hours of the pre-colonoscopy regimen and saying to my husband, "Huh, that's not so bad."

What's also not so bad is the entire procedure if you have the proper insurance. I highly recommend you do make sure the procedure is covered before you wander into the hospital because you want to be completely knocked out for an endoscopy and/or colonoscopy. Trust me on this one. Go sell a few pieces of jewelry to cover the general anesthesia if it's not covered. *Because someone is going to shove a tube with a camera down your throat and up your rectum.* You do NOT want to be awake for that. Also, you don't want to hear what everyone is saying about you in the procedure room as they get an intimate look at areas of your body that process food into waste.

When I finally did wake up, none the wiser about the violations that had just taken place, I learned that I did indeed have celiac disease. Shockingly, this was a relief that perhaps you too can relate to when you finally figure out what the heck is going on with your body. Because my first thought was *Thank god it wasn't cancer or Crohn's*. Sorry, Crohn's people, again—I wish I could wave a magic wand over your insides. But then I had some even more urgent thoughts, ones that you may have as well.

Questions you may have, and should totally ask, when you wake up from the anesthesia:

- Can I eat cake?

- Can I eat cupcakes?

- What about those mini cupcakes?

- Not even on my birthday?

- Who the hell do you think you are?

- Is that even a *real* college? Or did you get that degree from a
  Cracker Jack box?

- Can I eat Cracker Jack?

- Did you leave your head up my butt while you were in there?

- Are you sure?

- Then you won't mind if I shove something up *your* butt?

Hopefully your GI doc will be as chill as mine and won't threaten to go back in while you're awake and "can really feel it."

It's shocking to discover you can't eat something that is basically everywhere and in everything you want to eat. Especially shocking because I honestly don't know if I had even *heard* of gluten at that point. Of course I was about to get intimately acquainted with that toxic beast. By intimately acquainted, I mean stalking it and bad-mouthing it to anyone who would listen, followed by lots of crying because I missed that awful gluten.

It's true that this whole procedure of the emptying of your bowels, being

By the Numbers

Approximately three million Americans have been diagnosed with celiac disease, and the working theory is that another two million are going around eating gluten willy-nilly and getting sick, without a diagnosis. There are twenty million Americans who are gluten intolerant, poor things. So there are quite a few of us here in the U.S.A. trying to get rid of the gluten in our lives. To help you get a visual of how many of us are out there shopping, talking back to waiters, and being generally aggressive about our food, here's how the gluten-free stack up to other populations in America.

There are more people who can't eat the devil gluten than:

- Juggalos at the annual Insane Clown Posse Gathering
- Voted for Ross Perot for president of the United States in 1992
- Breastfeed their baby until the age of one year. Not that it's any of your damn business.
- Know all the words to "Free Bird"

There are fewer people who can't eat the devil gluten than:

- Are "Single" on Facebook
- Ryan Gosling fans
- Voted for Michael Dukakis for president of the United States (who knew?)
- Have sung the chorus of "Sweet Caroline" loudly, while drunk, at a bar
- Have forgotten about singing "Sweet Caroline" loudly, while drunk, somewhere that they can't quite recall

knocked out, and having things shoved inside of you is unpleasant, but it is a necessary step to make sure you have celiac disease. Then you can rest easy knowing that you can never eat gluten again for the rest of your life. And that's how the procedure goes, unless you're one of those people who have celiac disease but never have any gastrointestinal problems. Oh, hell, you didn't realize that was a thing, did you?

What to Do If You're NOT Crapping Your Pants

Let's talk about *that* whackness. For some celiacs, or some people who simply react badly to consuming gluten, it's not the pooping that drives them to diagnosis. There are a whole host of non-gastrointestinal symptoms that are related to celiac disease, including dermatitis herpetiformis. After you say that five times fast, you're going to have an itchy, red rash to scratch, thanks to gluten. Even though you're not having diarrhea, constipation, or vomiting, if you have celiac you're just as unable to absorb the necessary nutrients and can still face all those fun diseases like cancer or osteoporosis if you do not get diagnosed and get on that gluten-free diet. Other symptoms of celiac that are non-gastro-related include:

- Depression
- Brain fog
- Anemia
- Joint pain/Arthritis
- Muscle cramps
- Mouth sores
- Acid reflux
- Dental and bone disorders
- Neuropathy (tingling in your extremities)
- Exhaustion and weakness
- Stunted growth

- Weight loss

- Fertility problems and miscarriage

- Anxiety (Aren't you getting anxious just reading this list?)

- Migraines

- Acne

- Eczema

So what I'm trying to say is, having celiac disease as well as gluten sensitivity is an amazing time, and you'll always be the life of the party.

Why Me?

If you're as self-indulgent as I am, you may be wondering why in the name of all things holy you wound up with this autoimmune disorder or allergic reaction, or intolerance, or whatever the heck it is that's going down in your intestines. Although historically the medical community believed this was a white person's disease—specifically people from the UK and wherever they colonized (which is a lot of places, *amiright?*)—celiac and gluten sensitivity has now been discovered on every continent. Which means we're not alone. Sure, you may be Irish, but you don't *have* to be to have sprue. Also, it's possible to have the genetic markers for the sprue but no symptoms for a very long time. Which is what happened to me, until one fateful day with a frozen pizza.

One theory I floated to my gastroenterologist and my nutritionist—that they both seemed to be on board with—was that my recent food poisoning had something to do with my current condition. Although no one was willing to go on record and confirm, I've heard anecdotes about food poisoning being the beginning of the end of a gluten-filled diet. In fact, if you want me to get all celebrity on you, *The View* cohost and token Republican, Elisabeth Hasselbeck, and I both have celiac, and we both had a major incident with food poisoning prior to getting all sick in our pants. See? Two ladies, one common thread.

Apparently we are not alone in that because there is a brand-spanking-new study that has shown a connection between gastroenteritis and celiac disease[3] wherein patients experience a bacterial intestinal infection twenty-four months prior to experiencing symptoms of celiac disease. Although more studies need to be done, this is the beginning of research that totally backs me up in my theory that had I skipped a poison pizza, I'd still be enjoying donuts. Because it is clear to me that I was eating the hell out of gluten, and never had any physical ailment as a result, before I wound up in the hospital with severe food poisoning. I also was incredibly lucky to have had two very healthy pregnancies before this particular hammer came down upon me, which is challenging for a celiac woman who wishes to reproduce. So there.

In the summer of 2009, right after my son was born, I was enjoying a frozen pizza with not one, not two, but THREE meats atop its crust. Within about an hour I was emptying my bowels and my stomach with such severity that I began to resemble an opiate addict detoxing on *Celebrity Rehab with Dr. Drew*. Which may be why the fine people at the Brooklyn emergency room I found myself in did not take me seriously and I almost died. My general practitioner determined that it was E. coli, or salmonella, or some kind of serious poisoning that came from meat. Since the only meat I had eaten (or the only three meats I had eaten) in several days had come from that nasty-ass pizza, I wrote a letter to Stouffer's. I got a check for $20 and some coupons for more Lean Cuisine products, and apparently the beginning of my celiac disease symptoms. A note to Lean Cuisine: If someone gets violently ill on your product, a coupon to eat it again may not sway him or her. Maybe.

I'm not sure whether to curse the day Mr. and Mrs. Stouffer conceived baby Stouffer, who then tried his hand at a leaner cuisine, or to thank them for helping me identify a potentially life-threatening disease. I'm going with cursing because this was most likely the trigger for my gastrointestinal symptoms, which just might have been dormant and thus allowing me to enjoy wedding cake instead of sitting in the back, cursing love. At the same time, I come from a family fairly riddled with autoimmune disorders, and celiac apparently is mine. Woo-hoo! Yet with any autoimmune disease, the whys

3 Reuters Health, July 4, 2012.

and hows are incredibly shady. This is why anyone with a weird autoimmune thing will experience intense frustration with getting a diagnosis and trying to find a treatment. But luckily for those of us getting diagnosed now, there is much more awareness and much less "This is so totally in your head. Take a Valium and call me next year." Not that I wouldn't mind a Valium when I'm at yet another school function that starts directly after work when I'm at maximum starvation and that serves only pasta and bread.

If you're one of those people who have gluten sensitivity, it's possible it took even longer for you to figure out what was bugging you. I've known people who were so sick they began the elimination diet in earnest, only to drop it after four days of eating air. I also wonder how many doctors who have prescribed the elimination diet have actually done it themselves because that is one ridiculous thing to do to yourself. If you've never been on the elimination diet, consider yourself lucky. Here's what you're not allowed to eat, in pursuit of what food is making your body miserable: dairy, eggs, gluten, corn, sulfites (wine! Ahhhhhh!), soy, citrus fruits, caffeine (again, ahhhhhhh!), and all processed foods. So enjoy that hunk of grass-fed meat for a few weeks 'cause that's all you can have. If you came to your gluten intolerance diagnosis in this manner, I salute you while thanking god for my violent illness so I didn't have to do this crazy diet.

There IS a super-duper silver lining to all of this (or so I keep telling myself): You have a disease that's 100 percent reversible if you do one thing. Yes, that one thing is to never eat gluten again for the rest of your life. And while that may suck, it's a heck of a lot better than having to medicate, receive blood transfusions, or organ transplants. Don't you feel better already? No?

Then come with me and figure out how you can turn that intolerant, allergic, or celiac frown upside down! It's time to bust up some gluten and dive into the gluten-free pool of deliciousness. No, I'm not kidding. You can have deliciousness without gluten. I swear on my mother's muffin pan.

Chapter Two

SO YOU CAN'T EAT

Gluten

ANYMORE

Y ou may be sitting at home right now with a steak and a head of broccoli. If so, good for you! *That's totally gluten-free.* Don't let anyone tell you it's weird to sit around with your food in your lap, massaging it gently and pondering life. You're off to a fantastic start. Although steak and broccoli do make a perfectly acceptable meal, at some point you're going to want to branch out. That means you're going to have to go grocery shopping. You're also going to have to take out a loan to buy lots of gluten-free substitutes. Because gluten-free food costs more to produce, what with its fancy clean machinery, low demand, weird grains, and with no gluten dripping all over the place. That cost, of course, is passed on to you. I'm just telling you because I don't want you to get sticker shock the first time you pick up your gluten-free crackers and gluten-free beer for the holiday weekend. Because nothing says "party" like crackers and beer! You are welcome. And here's where I give you the good news: Gluten-free food for the sick is tax deductible under medical expenses. What? That's right, gluten-free food is like your medicine now, people. So write that shizzle off.[4]

But before you go crazy like I did, don't race to your local health food

---

[4] Talk to your accountant to make this legal, not some lady writing a book with a curse word in the title.

store and buy up everything with a GF label and go home and make amaranth donuts, sorghum donuts, rice donuts, and gluten-free potato chip donuts. Stop and assess your new lifestyle. Yes, it is a lifestyle even if it's been forcibly imposed. Maybe you only need two varieties of gluten-free chocolate chip cookie dough. And probably one gluten-free brownie mix will do it for you. Oh, hell, what do I care? *Go crazy in the gluten-free aisle* (or shelf, as your store may not be with it just yet). It will be cathartic. Stock those cabinets with buckwheat noodles and gluten-free scone mix. Try your hand at recreating Chelsea Clinton's gluten-free wedding cake! Why not? But just in case you don't want to spend your entire paycheck on gluten-free options that you wind up throwing in the trash, maybe keep reading.

Your new diet food can be categorized in two ways: the naturally gluten-free and the not-at-all naturally gluten-free but it is now thanks to science. I feel the urge to tell you that naturally gluten-free food is going to be the better choice. However, you're going to want some of that not-natural stuff as well *because it's delicious.* Not as delicious as that Twix bar you can no longer have, but food companies are making great strides, and I honestly expect the Twix people to present me with a delicious gluten-free version any day now. I'm waiting.

Here's how it all breaks down.

Naturally Gluten-Free Foods That Are Your New Best Friends

You'll be shocked at all the foods that contain the devil gluten. But since you probably never paid one second of attention to gluten before, you might be just as shocked at the quantity of foods that do not naturally contain gluten. These foods are your very best friends. You don't have to specially prepare them or mix them while crying because the xanthan gum is making your fingers all weirdly slippery. (Oh, you'll find out all about xanthan gum, don't you worry.) You can just pick them off a tree, slice them off an animal, or milk them from a cow, and you're good to go. That's why that broccoli-and-steak dinner was such a great idea. Good job for thinking of that!

Just like all those people who write books with rules on how to eat healthy and avoid the grocery store glut, if you stick to the aisles around the sides of the store you'll probably be safe. I mean, not totally safe. There's sausage out there, after all. But here are the safest, and chilliest, sections of the grocery store to get your gluten-free eat on:

- Butcher/Fish counter
- Produce (that's fruits and vegetables for you former fast-food devotees)
- Dairy

Bring your sweater.

Meat Is the Word

Meat and fish, in its natural form, is totally gluten-free. Yes, even grass-fed beef. (That was an actual question ℓ someone had—don't make fun.) Please note that packaged meat is not in its natural form. Meat with "natural flavors" is not at all natural, and you must find out what those flavors are made of because a lot of times those flavors are made out of gluten. The good news is, if you're shopping for cuts of meat with the help of your butcher, so long as no one has slathered a marinade or bread crumbs all over it, you're safe to buy out the entire store and go home and eat it. That's right, I just gave you permission to go on a meat gorge. Go crazy! Oh, except for that one super-delicious meat.

The delicious, yet deadly, sausage I mentioned earlier, for example. You don't have to give up sausage completely (thank you, gluten-loving Jesus!), you just have to do one of two things: Buy gluten-free sausage or make sausage at home yourself. Sometimes the latter is actually easier because people love to fill up tube meats with other business that, although delicious, will make the gluten intolerant keel over. Even if you're buying sausage from your friendly neighborhood butcher, he might be using a wheat-based casing around that pure sausage meat. Ahem, I said "pure." Obviously the same goes for hot dogs. Do not eat a dog until you've checked its credentials. This is good advice in any situation. For both sausage and hot dogs, I have found that Applegate does a damn good job of keeping the mixed meat gluten-free. It's also organic and anti-antibiotic, which is only helpful to those of us with issues. Yes, I just strongly implied that you should go organic. Don't hate.

Why Go Organic?

I'm not here to tell you that you can only put organic quinoa in your body from now on (though someone will tell you that, you can bet on it), but I will say this—the less junk in your food, the less likely you'll wind up on the bowl. Organic produce, dairy, meat, even organic processed food is simply better for your body's digestive system. The less crap up in there, the better. You're sensitive now; act like it.

Organic means no synthetic pesticides used on your food, no human sewage fertilizer used (ewwwww! Now you'll *never* eat nonorganic, right?), no antibiotics used in animals, and strict separation of organic and nonorganic crops grown with the help of chemicals. It is hoped all organic products will begin to also be labeled as non-GMO foods, and GMO foods will soon be labeled as such. That's genetically modified organisms, for those of you keeping score at home, and that means food that has been messed with, and not for the better. Say it with me: "No more GMOs! No more GMOs!" Ready to storm the castle? Let's have some organic gluten-free chocolate first, shall we?

To recap: Spend the extra and go organic, just so you know you're not getting poisonous compounds along with your grapes. Your beat-up stomach will thank you. Unless you can't find it, you can't afford it, or some other reason like "Seriously? Why are you telling me what to do? You promised not to tell me what to do!" It's OK, you do what you've got to do to stay gluten-free and able to pay your rent. I'm just saying organic is where it's at.

Produce

It's a fact that you can eat as many greens as you'd like and ingest zero gluten. That also goes for oranges, reds, purples, and whatever other colors you find in your fruits and vegetables. In their original form, fruits and vegetables are gluten-free. Just don't add any gluten to that business, and you'll be good. Sadly, this also means "pie." You cannot add pie to your fruit and still be eating gluten-free. Unless, of course, you use one of my gluten-free pie recipes! I *told* you this book was going to be good.

Really, any produce is great for you, and of course, most of it should be organic. See page 33 for organic diatribe. If it's not available to you, or it's just too dang expensive, at the very least buy these "dirty dozen[5]" foods in the organic section. These are the fruits and vegetables most easily contaminated by pesticides:

- Peaches
- Apples
- Sweet bell peppers
- Nectarines, imported
- Strawberries
- Celery
- Lettuce
- Potatoes
- Grapes
- Spinach
- Cucumbers
- Blueberries

---

5 Environmental Working Group

I don't mean to harp on the organic thing. For those of you who read the study out of Stanford that said organic is not more healthy than nonorganic, remember that I'm talking to you—the people with food issues. It's not that you're looking for a healthier apple with more vitamins; instead you're looking for an apple that hasn't been sprayed with chemicals or crossbred with an almond that could wreak havoc on your sensitive gut. I just want to make sure you know what's up with your groceries. I'm also not saying one can live on produce alone, but if you're like, "Oh my god! Everything has gluten! I can't eat one damn thing!!!" remember: produce. It's your gluten-free buddy. You can always roll that orange in sugar and/or beef if you're really feeling panicked. In fact, that's one of my recipes! (*Editor's note: It's totally not one of her recipes; that is disgusting.*)

Cheese, Beautiful Cheese

I worked hard to earn the nickname "The Dairy Queen," which is why it was such a shock to me when I heard that oftentimes gluten and dairy problems go together. I was even more shocked when someone implied that perhaps it would be a great idea for me to go dairy-free. And imagine how shocked he was when he wound up in a headlock, between my armpit and my bosom.

I love dairy. I love cheese, butter, and cheesy-butter. I think milkshakes are the nectar of the gods, and I wouldn't kick a fro-yo out of my bed. For those of us who are on restricted diets, it's these other comfort foods that will get us through. Mine happens to be dairy. You'll find your own, but if you're searching: May I suggest dairy? If you must be dairy-free, allow me to offer my most sincere condolences and suggest you skip right over to the next section. Also, check out my vegan recipes because they are also delicious. No, I'm not kidding.

If you're lucky like me, however, you'll get much enjoyment by bulking up on almost every single dairy product. Notice I said almost. Although a recent report came out saying blue cheese is now OK for the gluten intolerant, I've heard many murmurings that the opposite is true. Apparently there's this thing about the bread mold that makes the blue business all up on the cheese. Bread that has gluten. Gluten that hates you. I'm sure by the time this book winds up on shelves and somewhere in cyberspace, someone will have tossed out another opinion on the elusive blue cheese. So unless you think you'll die without it, skip it until you hear otherwise. Remember, there's always Gouda. Here's where I remind you again—go organic and antibiotic free. You really, really, really don't want weird stuff in your dairy because it travels through your body and turns right into man boobs.

I would be remiss in not pointing out that not all foods found in the dairy section of your grocery are created equal. Of course cheese, yogurt, milk, and butter in the purest form are all naturally gluten-free. But dairy is so damn good, people love to get in there and muck it up. That's because they're just jealous. You've seen that yogurt with the M&Ms and granola? If only they'd stopped at the M&Ms, you'd be safe. Granola, however, is a killer. Every processed food—even those made from beloved dairy—must be scrutinized. It was perhaps one of the saddest days of my life when my go-to spinach-artichoke dip was marked off my faves list due to the words "Made in a facility that processes wheat." Sure, it's possible that wheat-processing machine never touched my dip, but who knows? Not me. At least, not until I wound up bent over the toilet bowl.

And that's the thing about going gluten-free: Some of us are more sensitive than others. If you happen to have celiac disease, or just happen to be really, really, sensitive, you can't even eat gluten-free food that has interacted with gluten. By interacting I mean made in the same mixer, factory, or even kitchen. Which brings us to the conversation I've been dreading: the cross-contamination discussion.

Cross-Contamination: Buyer Beware

Whether you're dining out, dining in, grocery shopping, or Dumpster diving, you've got to take notice of where your gluten-free food has been. You are now a gluten-free food stalker, and you must embrace this creepy fact.

Sometimes identifying gluten-free contaminated food is as obvious as trying to pry that Brie off a baguette, other times it's totally unclear and no, you do not understand why you cannot have that gluten-free pizza that was made on the same surface as a gluten-filled pizza. Especially since not one single ingredient is gluten. The thing is, gluten is sticky. If you put a croissant down on a plate, some croissant-y gluten will stick to it. So don't even think about licking that plate in hopes of tasting croissant again. Trust me on that one.

The bummer of the situation is, if you pick up a food that has also been processed on the same machinery—or sometimes in the same facility—as wheat, you can get glutened. That's why the little gluten-free symbol on packaged foods is so hard to get. That business has to be clean. This is also why if you make a (gluten-free, natch) dip and serve it up with gluten-free bagel chips alongside gluten-filled bagel chips, you're going to get glutened. Other people's dipping of the gluten into your dip will wind up in your body. I know! It's the most annoying thing about eating gluten-free. But it's not quite as annoying as pooping out your insides every five minutes. Some more fun examples of cross-contamination include:

• You use the same pasta pot to make your gluten-free pasta right after you made that gluten-filled mac and cheese for the kids.

• You simply scrape that gravy off your mashed potatoes and move on. Not so fast. Unless you're running to the bathroom.

• Someone came over to your house when you were out of town and put his chicken fingers in your oven and on your pan. And now your pan has those stuck-on crunchies attached to its surface like forever. Not that I'm mad or anything, Aaron.

• You pick out the gluten-free Rice Chex from the Chex Mix that includes gluten-filled pretzels and gluten-filled soy sauce.

• Same mixing spoon used for two very different recipes. Obviously one has gluten in it. You get where I'm going here, right?

• You make out with someone who just ate a piece of chocolate cake. (Although honestly, why would you kiss someone who is flaunting his cake-eating abilities in front of you? Plus—get a room.)

All of these examples, as well as those that are clearly labeled on your dip, are ways to get sick even when you think you're eating gluten-free. These reasons are also why some people will tell you to get rid of all of your pots and pans and start over with gluten-free cookware. These same people will suggest you march into everyone's kitchen and demand to see how the food is prepared. Although I appreciate this rigid approach to your health, and it's totally true that it will save your stomach from many woes, I will tell you that I do none of those things.

I do have one pot and strainer that is dedicated to anything gluten-related, and I try to keep the other ones (which were used to cook up big ol' pots of gluten before my diagnosis) clean and gluten-free at all times. I also tossed my wooden spoons and wooden cutting boards because those wooden tools like to hoard gluten. Yet I've also been known to indulge in a bean dip that was made in the same factory as gluten. Many times. Come on, it's yummy, yummy bean dip! Did I get sick? No. Could something have happened inside me that I was not aware of? Of course. In fact, it most surely has. Which is why I will now make the announcement that I'm a risk-taker, a rebel. It's certainly easier for me to find a restaurant to meet up with friends when I have this laissez-faire attitude about cross-contamination. And it's definitely helpful in that I didn't throw out all of my wedding gifts and restock my kitchen once I was diagnosed. But you know what happened to me at my follow-up visit? Flat villi. You don't want that, so listen up.

You've got to make your own choices on how stringent you're going to be regarding cross-contamination, and every doctor will tell you to be ever vigilant. But remember, unless you're in your own kitchen, you can't control everything. Even gluten-free menus are at the mercy of the person preparing your food. Just by going to someone else's kitchen you're taking a chance. Either you're willing to do that, or you are not. Hey, it's cool either way. I understand that my lack of willingness to be a crazed harpy when I walk into a restaurant could cost me a centimeter or two of villi. It's a chance I take, but not one I recommend for everyone. Or hell, anyone. Hence, my "buyer beware" warning. But if you're serious about keeping gluten out of your gut, you've really got to be intense about this. And sometimes, intense means totally annoying. (See Chapter 4.) But hey, who are we kidding? Gluten-free people are already annoying by simply existing. At least according to assholes everywhere.

So Where Do I Find the Doughnuts?

I'm so sorry, but you can't have real doughnuts anymore. Correction: You can have doughnuts that actually taste like cake. Those fluffy, crispy-skinned doughnuts are really not in your future. But I do have a rad recipe for beignets! Although not as poufy as a Krispy Kreme, they do have some air up in them. And they're French! But never fear, in addition to the amazoids recipes found here, there are a ton of gluten-free desserts out there for you to grab and go when you're at the store. You can still have super-delicious desserts that will add just as many (or more!) pounds onto your ass as those with delicious gluten. It's a win/win. Here are a few of my favorite things:

- Ice cream, gelato, sorbet—So long as there aren't any cookie pieces or other add-ins that are covered in gluten, enjoy!

- Flan—Naturally gluten-free, naturally fat-adding. YUM.

- M&Ms—You may find yourself living on these wonders because you can find them anywhere.

- Chocolate-covered almonds—Or any nut, really. Yes, I'm going to say it. Go nuts!

- French macarons—Most of them, anyway. Occasionally some will have gluten, so always ask. (You may be thinking: *Macarons, really? Where, pray tell, do I find macarons in my small province?* Macarons are the hot new "it" dessert, replacing your local cupcake joint as I type. They'll be there, and they will be delicious.)

- Meringues—Fluffy balls of sugar with no gluten. What's not to like?

- Pudding—Not all pudding is created equal, but most brands and flavors are totally gluten-free. That goes for mousse too, which is just fancy pudding.

- Jell-O—Try the many flavors of pudding's cousin from the wrong side of the tracks, Jell-O. You can even enjoy them as a shot! (See the recipes.)

A Short Conversation About Flour

While we're on the topic of making delicious sweets, let's have a frank discussion about gluten-free flour, the basis of most great sweet things. Unlike the dark ages of every day before about four years ago, there are five million gluten-free flour options available to you. It's confusing. You can, and should, experiment with all of these grain flours that are gluten-free, like sorghum, brown rice, tapioca, quinoa, potato, millet, and the new kid on the block, green banana. (Although I'm not experimenting with green banana flour because that is just *weird*.) The idea behind mixing it up with different grain flours is you'll get a nutritional powerhouse by eating healthy grain flours rather than grabbing your basic gluten-free all-purpose flour that usually contains rice flour, cornstarch, potato starch, and maybe xanthan gum. This is a great idea. But let me tell you how this is going to go down. You'll buy all of these exotic flours, experiment once or twice, and abandon them in the back of your cabinet where they'll grow stale or be invaded by weevils and freak you out for life. That's just unhygienic, and quite frankly I don't even know if bugs are gluten-free. OK, bugs *are* totally gluten-free. Still, skip that step and grab the all-purpose. Let's talk about those!

Cup4Cup by Thomas Keller—I made the most amazing Christmas cookies using Cup4Cup Flour, and that's one reason I worship at the altar of Thomas Keller. When you use Cup4Cup gluten-free flour you also don't have to add xanthan gum. So when you look at my recipes, omit the xanthan gum if you're in possession of this fancy flour. However, there's no need to go all fancy-pants when you're battering your mozzarella sticks. Save this white gold for when it really matters, and you're feeling wealthy.

King Arthur's Gluten-Free Multi-Purpose Flour—There's a reason King Arthur's gluten-free multi-purpose flour has a recipe for popovers on the box. Because King Arthur's G-F M-P flour can be used to make some effing delicious popovers. This is a fantastic go-to for just about everything else as well. I've actually (knock on wood) never had anything turn out badly when using King Arthur's multi-purpose gluten-free flour. You do have to add xanthan gum if you're using Art's mix, but you'll always have a stash of that in your cabinets anyway now that you're a mutant.

Bob's Red Mill All-Purpose Gluten-Free Baking Flour—Bob is adorable and from Portland, Oregon. Do you need another reason? OK, here's one: BRM is committed to high-quality and safe products. They rock. Also, they make that xanthan gum I was talking about.

Better Batter Seasoned Flour Mix—If you're frying, this is the way to go. It's like Better Batter knows that what we really want, as gluten-haters, is that thick crunchy coating on our chicken/deep-fried Kool-Aid/broccoli. They are truly mind readers for the gluten-free. Better Batter's cup-for-cup all-purpose flour is also the bomb when you're baking, and you can skip that xanthan gum too.

Some people don't like using the exact cup-for-cup substitutions that are offered by Better Batter and Cup4Cup, but I've had consistent—and delicious—results using these mixtures. In fact, for the most part when I whip up something using either of these direct substitution flours, it's even better than using a mixture of other grain flours plus xanthan gum.

I'm thinking it's time I explained what xanthan gum is all about and why it keeps butting into every conversation. The thing about gluten is that it's incredibly sticky. Once you remove gluten from your baking equation, you've got a lack of sticky situation on your hands. Xanthan gum is a thickening agent in many foodstuffs, from salad dressings to sauces, and it also acts as the sticky when you're using gluten-free flours. Say you have a thing against the letter X; there's also guar gum. Both of these gums are gluten-free and used for the sole purpose of making food stable. Arrowroot is another thickening and sticky agent some chefs add to gluten-free single-grain flours, but it is incredibly expensive. Xanthan gum doesn't have a taste, but wow, does it feel funny. Thank goodness it doesn't feel funny in your mouth because then we'd never eat it and we'd be walking around without gluten-free cake. Xanthan gum gets weird once it comes into contact with liquid; it starts to feel like you're putting on a pair of silky gloves when you wash your hands after handling. But this is the least of your worries when it comes to the unpleasantness of gluten intolerance.

As you read this, there are a zillion other people developing gluten-free all-purpose flours. Experiment and find out how you get the best results in the easiest way possible. Although I'm all for trying every different combination of gluten-free goodness in order to find muffin nirvana, some night you're really just going to need to throw something in flour and deep-fry that sucker within an inch of its gluten-free life. It shouldn't be tougher than your high school chemistry class to make deep-fried goodness. I recommend making life easier and going all-purpose.

Sneaky A-Hole Foods That Have Gluten Even Though You'd Never Know It by Looking

Here's some more bad news, my friends. Gluten is a sneaky bastard. Sometimes you're all "Wow, this gluten-free meal is delicious—oh, damn." It happens to the best of us, and you live and you learn. Just so you don't have as many living-and-learning accidents in your pants as I did, I'm going to fill you in on those not-obvious glutenous foods that are no longer allowed in your gut.

Soy sauce—I don't get this, and I never will. But the sneakiest of all is the soy sauce. Because you don't exactly get that wheat feel when you're dining on sushi. Luckily there is a wheat-free tamari you can buy and carry with you when you head out for rolls. Of course, you have to ask if the plate of raw fish you're about to enjoy already has soy sauce dripping from its shiny loins. For some of you, this is an easy one. You're thinking, "I hate sushi!" Well, my picky friends, soy sauce is also found in marinades, salad dressings, and teriyaki sauce, making it the sneakiest gluten of all. What this means for you is that when you're over at a friend's house or at a restaurant, you have to explain the whole soy sauce thing. Then people will be like, "Wait, can you have tofu?" Because soy sauce sounds exactly like "soy," and people will be confused. Yes, you can have soy products of any kind, so long as they are not dripping in soy sauce. Annoying, I know.

WTF, Triticale?

We're all clear on what wheat, rye, and barley are when we gulp them down. If you're like me, when you heard that gluten intolerants cannot eat triticale you thought, *What in the hell is triticale? A club drug?* Worse. Triticale is the unholy marriage of rye and wheat. Why people felt the need to merge these two grains is beyond me, but I'm sure someone had a good reason. And that good reason was surely cash money. Regardless, here's where you can find triticale, and so here is what you must avoid. Also, look for triticale on cereal labels—especially cereals not made in the United States, because apparently triticale is more of an international crop and not found as frequently in the U.S.A. And so long as no one starts trading their Levi's for triticale seed, we Americans should be OK if we keep our eyes peeled.

• Cereal—Kashi Seven Whole Grain Blend, Bob's Red Mill Triticale Hot Cereal, and more
• Bob's Red Mill—Triticale Flour & Triticale Berries
• *Star Trek's* "The Trouble with Tribbles"—Seriously, they talked about triticale in that episode. I'm pretty sure you can't get glutened from watching *Star Trek,* but we never can be too careful, can we?

Oats—Oatmeal seemed like an excellent breakfast alternative to me when I was diagnosed with the celiac. No more Cap'n Crunch meant it was time for me to grow up. However, oats can bug a celiac like nobody's business. This is for a few reasons. One, some facilities cut their oats with flour. *Phhhhhpt.* Two, some gluten-intolerant folks find oats to be irritating as well.

Just to be safe, you should buy "pure, uncontaminated oats," and the package must be marked. Even then, only moderate amounts (½ cup to ¾ cup of such oats) are advised. I highly recommend you go out and get these pure oats; otherwise, you'll never be able to make my delicious gluten-free double chocolate oatmeal cookies. (See recipes.)

Soups—How did that yummy soup get so thick? Gluten. You know what else gets glutened to make them thick? Marinades, gravies, salad dressings, and sauces. Yes, even the next one.

Enchilada sauce—Yeah, I didn't even think this was a thing. It's a sauce, made from peppers and tomatoes. However, as I discovered, some enchilada sauce also has chicken broth, so vegetarians are not safe either. Let this be the lesson to all sensitive types: Any food that has a barcode must be considered suspect.

Play-Doh—If you were like me, you totally ate Play-Doh as a kid. Oh, you didn't? Well, don't start now because it has gluten in it.

Beer—Maybe beer is not so sneaky because it seemed to me that everyone warned me off having a cold one when I was first diagnosed. (Was it something I did?) But you may not automatically think of beer as having gluten. It does. Don't drink it. Unless it's gluten-free beer, but some of those even sneak some gluten inside, so read that label and/or call that beer company.

Communion Wafers—Sorry, religious folks who partake in the body of Christ, but you're going to be benched. Ask your priest or minister about providing an alternative or risk the wrath of the Lord.

Dextrin—What is this, you may ask? It's a sneaky starch that's used as a thickener and in medications. Yep, it's got gluten.

Baking Powder—Seriously, how annoying is that? Look for the gluten-free label on that staple.

Skinny Vanilla Lattes—Yep, learned that the hard way. Asshole mermaid.

Stamps and Envelopes—Hahahahahahaha. As if you use those anymore.

Vitamins and Medication—This one is a doozy. You need vitamins to make sure your new gluten-free self is getting all of the nutrients your sensitive body requires. Yet some vitamins and medications have gluten. Dang it! As for any medication you're taking, don't risk just reading the ingredients list, also ask the pharmacist. If s/he seems clueless, call the manufacturer.

Seriously, you don't want to give up normal good-tasting pizza just to get glutened by your cold medicine. Don't rely on a generic of a trusted medication either. I found myself getting glutened repeatedly by my generic Tylenol because the brand name is gluten-free. Turns out some of those generics (Safeway brand, I'm looking at you) throw some wheat starch in there without telling us, or rather, without a warning label. Never assume; you know what they say about that.

Malt—Whether it's that delicious one from the *shoppe* or the weird one at Long John Silver's, anything with the word "malt" is now forbidden because malt usually means barley malt.

Mustard—Not all mustard, but some types are made with ale. That's beer, if you're an American. Again, you've gotta read that label and/or call the company. I know! Your phone bill is getting ridiculous.

Licorice—And just as I moved to the land of Red Vines. This also goes for licorice flavoring.

Lunch Meat—Some brands of cold cuts, like Boar's Head, pride themselves on being gluten-free. Others are chock full of fillers. Fillers with gluten. Is your phone ready for more action? Call 'em.

Touching Bagels—OK, most of you know that you can't eat bagels anymore. Obvious gluten source, am I right? I discovered the hard way ("the hard way" means pooping like crazy with a house full of guests I had just fed breakfast) that even touching a bagel can trigger an attack. I don't know if it's because bagels are jam-packed with gluten ~~or I licked my hands after~~ or have a secret weapon that shoots bagelness into your bloodstream just by standing near, but we can no longer have bagels in our house that could possibly come into contact with any part of my body. That's right, *any* part. (Note: Since you have to actually ingest gluten to get sick, I certainly touched a bagel and licked my hand because I'm disgusting like that. So just don't touch a bagel, in case of the licking. If you must touch a bagel, wash your hands and lick away.)

Your takeaway here is this: Anything that comes with a label or in a package must be treated as suspect. If it is not food in its purest form (and its purest form is not wheat, rye, barley, or triticale), you've got to figure out exactly what was used in the making of said food. Everyone has been lying to us about salad being good for us because salad has so many places to hide the gluten. Gluten is a fiend and must be ferreted out. Now you know why some people only eat steak and broccoli.

Do I Have Cancer?
And Other Joys of Being a Celiac

If you're diagnosed with celiac, you may have other things to worry about if you don't banish gluten from your presence. How much do we really need to worry, on a scale of "Starting a bucket list RIGHT NOW" to "Really? So I have a better chance of marrying a terrorist?" Well, if you cut gluten out of your diet you can dramatically decrease the chances of your developing one of these horrible diseases that are complications resulting from untreated celiac. In fact, the best way to keep these diseases far away from your body is to go gluten-free and stay that way. Then you've got a better chance of being killed in a car accident. This is the feel-good part of the book, obviously. Ready to be scared straight?

- Malnutrition
- Anemia
- Osteoporosis
- Rickets
- Lymphoma
- Bowel cancer
- Peripheral neuropathy
- Seizures
- Thyroid disease